BREAST SURGERY

CLINICAL PATHWAY

Prepared by
Dr. Badria Eid Al-Johani

01 July, 2015

Copyright © 2015 by Eid & Otto Internationale
All rights reserved. No unauthorized reproductions are permitted
Without express written approval from Eid & Otto Internationale

Breast surgery clinical pathway

Written by

Dr. Badria Eid Al-Johani
Consultant General Surgery
Consultant Breast & Endocrine Surgery
Riyadh, Kingdom of Saudi Arabia

Copyright © 2015 by Eid & Otto Internationale
All rights reserved. No part of this book may be reproduced without written consent from Eid & Otto Internationale

ISBN: 978-0-9909322-2-2

Printed on Demand by Createspace.com
Distributed by Amazon and Amazon international affiliates

Contact Eid & Otto Internationale
info@eid-otto.com

Visit us
http://www.eid-otto.com

Eid & Otto Internationale
1712 Pioneer Ave, Suite 670
Cheyenne, WY, 82001
USA

1 (469)-208-3100

Breast Surgery Clinical Pathway
Copyright © 2015 by Eid & Otto Internationale
All rights reserved. No unauthorized reproductions are permitted
Without express written approval from Eid & Otto Internationale

Breast surgery clinical pathway

TABLE OF CONTENTS

INTRODUCTION	3
GENERAL INFORMATION	4
COMPONENTS OF PATHWAY	5
CLINCAL PATHWAY OF BREAST SURGERY UNIT	7
CLINCAL PATHWAY ON SPECIAL POPULATIONS	
PREGNANCY	16
HIGH RISK	17
EMERGENCY SURGERY	18
OUTSIDE RESIDENTS	18
SURGICAL COMPLICATIONS	
HEMATOMA AND BLEEDING	19
WOUND INFECTION AND SKIN NECROSIS	20
SEROMA	20
CHRONIC PAIN	21
DEEP VENOUS THROBOSIS	21
CLINICAL RESPONSIBLITIES	
RESIDENTS	22
SPECIALISTS	24
WEEKLY SCHEDULE FOR BREAST SURGERY UNIT	26
DOCTOR AND PATIENT RELATIONS AND CONFIDENTIALITY	27
UNDERGRADUATE AND POST GRADUATE TRAINING	29
CHECKLIST	
BREAST DISEASES HISTORY	31
BREAST PHYSICAL EXAM	32
COMBINED BREAST CLINC ORDERS	33
PRE-OPERATIVE BREAST SURGERY ORDERS	34
OPERATIVE NOTE	35
POST OPERATIVE INSTRUCTION FOR MASTECTOMY	36
POST OPERATIVE INSTRUCTION FOR SKIN SPARING MASTECTOMY	38
POST OPERATIVE INSTRUCTION FOR LUMPECTOMY	39
DAILY PROGRESS NOTE	56
DRAIN CARE	57
BREAST TEAM ROUNDS	
PRE OPERATIVE BREAST TEAM ROUND	58
POST OPERATIVE BREAST TEAM	59
DISCHARGE	60
APPOINTMENTS	60
POST DISCHARGE ASSESMENT FOR WOUND CARE NURSE	61
WOUND CARE	63

Copyright © 2015 by Eid & Otto Internationale
All rights reserved. No unauthorized reproductions are permitted
Without express written approval from Eid & Otto Internationale

Breast surgery clinical pathway

INTRODUCTION

Breast cancer is the most common cancer among females, and the incidence is steadily increasing worldwide.

Due to the increasing the complexity of breast cancer treatment it is of paramount importance to develop a structured care in order to avoid non-consistent management of patients. Clinical pathways can be used to improve efficiency and quality of care. They also aim to re-center the focus on the patient's overall journey, rather than the contribution of each specialty or caring function independently.

GENERAL INFORMATION

Aim:

Our aim is to produce clinical pathway for all patients undergoing breast surgery in order to optimize patient's recovery in our breast surgery unit.

Targeted populations;

All adult patients who undergo breast surgery

Users;

This pathway is intendant to be used by all staff who are involved in management of breast surgery.

Outcomes of interest;

Decrease post-operative complications; enhance patient's recovery, decrease patients Stay and increase patient's satisfactions.

COMPONENTS OF SURGICAL PATHWAY

1. Pre-operative component

   1.1 counseling and education;

   1.2 Admission;

2. Peri-operative component

   2.1 pre surgery support;

   2.2 surgery support

   2.3 Post surgery support

3. Post-operative component

   3.1Discharge

   3.2 post discharge support

4. Follow-up

Table 1. SUMMARY OF CLINICAL PATHWAY OF BREAST SURGERY UNIT

Guideline	Component	Time	Location	Note
Pre-operative	Counseling and Education	First clinic visit	Combined Breast clinic	• history /physical exam checklist • Imaging • Biopsy/review pathology slides
		5th day	Tumor board	• Conference checklist • Management plan
		10th -12th day **or** after Neoadjuvant therapy	Surgical breast clinic	• Surgical plan and booking
			Patient counselor	• Patient education and counseling
			Anesthesia clinic	• Pre-operative anesthesia
	Admission	Within one month of first visit	Surgical ward	• Admission note • Preoperative orders checklist
Peri-operative	Pre surgery support	Day 0	Surgical ward	• Team round checklist • Lymphoscintigraphy • Wire localization
	Surgery support	Day 0	Theater	• Positioning • Pathology report • Operative note checklist • Post-operative orders checklist
	Post-surgery support		Surgical ward	• Team round checklist • Pain control • Mobilization
Post-operative	Discharge	Day 1	Surgical ward	• Team round checklist • Wound &Drain care • Appointments and Medications • Patient reassurance • accommodation and flight tickets • Physiotherapy
	Post discharge support	Day 3	Wound care nurse clinic	• Wound dressing • drain care • patient reassurance
		Day 5		• Drain check for removal • Wound dressing
			Tumor board	• Appointment for adjuvant therapy
Follow-up		Day 15	Breast Surgery clinic	• check wound • discus pathology result • Follow-up after 3-6 months.
			Wound care clinic	• Wound care • Confirm drain removal
			Physiotherapy clinic	• physiotherapy
		Day 22	Physiotherapy clinic	• physiotherapy
			Wound care nurse clinic	• Clips removal • wound care
		Day 30		• Confirm the Wound is healed. • Drain and clips are removed. • Discharge

CLINICAL PATHWAY OF BREAST SURGERY UNIT:

Components of clinical pathway for breast surgery can be categorized into pre-operative, peri-operative and post-operative, see table 1.

1. Pre-operative components:

Pre-operative component starts from the first day of the patient's visit to the breast unit clinic until the patient is admitted into the ward for surgery.

1.1 Patient counseling and education:

Recommendation;
a) *All patients who have breast cancer are seen in the combined breast clinic.*
b) *The combined breast clinic checklist is completed by the multidisciplinary team (surgery, oncology and radiotherapy).*
c) *Each patient from the combined clinic is discussed in tumor board meeting; a consensus management plan is formulated and recorded.*
d) *For Patients who are suitable for surgical treatment or who have finished Neoadjuvant systemic therapy, the surgical options are discussed in the breast surgery clinic in a very clear manner with all possible complications and alternative procedures including reconstructive options. Upon obtaining consent from the patient for the intended procedure, the patient will be scheduled for surgery within one month or 3 weeks from the last dose of Neoadjuvant chemotherapy.*
e) *All surgical patients will be informed about what they will expect during the course of hospital stay including surgery, post-operative recovery, diet, ambulation, drain, and duration of hospital stay. Written information about her disease, surgical procedures, and complications will be provided to each patient.*
f) *All patients will have a complete Evaluation of risk factors will be controlled; (Hypertension, Diabetes, COPD, Asthma, Cardiac disease, Malnutrition and Anemia) by pre-anesthesia clinic and the involved services.*

Combined breast clinic:

A rapid diagnosis of cancer breast is achieved. Close coordination and communication between the breast surgeon, medical oncologist, radiation physician, radiologist, histopathologist, and breast care nurse and clerical staff.

All patients are seen first by breast coordinator, who will take a brief personal data including contacting numbers, and then the patient will be seen by the multidisciplinary team (medical oncologist, surgeon, radiation therapy) with triple assessment are achieved.

Breast Tumor conference:

The weekly breast tumor conference is an integral part of the breast cancer care pathway and has improved the quality of care for all breast cancer patients. Each patient, from combined clinic and post-operative cases are discussed and a consensus management plan is formulated and recorded. The multidisciplinary team approach recognizes that each breast cancer patient is unique in terms of disease characteristics, psychological and social issues, and requires an individualized treatment plan. The meetings also have an educational value for Specialists, surgical residents and trainees. Additionally, patients suitable for national and international trials are identified at the multidisciplinary team meeting. The patients are contacted by a breast care coordinator with an appointment in the appropriate breast cancer clinic within one week.

Breast Cancer Clinic:

Following the multidisciplinary team meeting, the patients are ideally seen in the appropriate breast cancer clinic to discuss the results of the diagnostic and staging workup .A comprehensive plan regarding the management of their disease is presented in each patient.

Patients who are suitable for surgical treatment or who finished Neoadjuvant systemic therapy, surgical options are discussed in the breast surgery clinic in a very clear manner with all possible complications and alternative procedures.

1.2 Patient's admission:

Recommendation:

a) The surgeon will confirm the date of surgery with the patient one week before.

b) All scheduled procedures are confirmed with operating room scheduling and the plastic surgeon one week before the procedure.

c) Patients are admitted through the admission office where a bed is booked for her/him.

d) Personal hygiene kit is given to each patient, including the hospital robe and slippers, toothbrush and paste.

e) Patients are advised to take a shower and clean both breast and axilla with antiseptic gel on the day of surgery.

f) If the patient has axillary hair, a hair clipper (not blade) is used for removal to avoid skin wound on the morning of surgery.

g) If admission occurs during working hours, the breast team is called in to complete the admission notes and preoperative orders (admission note checklist, pre-operative order checklist). If after working hours, this is completed by the on-call team.

h) All patients who are planned for reconstructive surgery are seen by the plastic surgeon before surgery.

2. Peri-operative components:

Peri-operative component is started on the day of surgery and lasts until the patient is shifted to the ward after surgery.

2.1 Pre-surgery support:

Recommendation:

a) Patients who need a wire localization procedure or lymphoscintigraphy for sentinel lymph node biopsy are sent to the appropriate department at 0730 A.M. Arrangements should be made with breast radiology and nuclear medicine one day before surgery, and the patient should be in the room within 30 minutes before OR call to avoid OR delay when they call for the next patient.

b) All patients' belongings, including jewelry, hair clips, mobile, credit cards or money should be kept with her/his supporter.

c) Avoid unnecessary mobilization for patients with a wire localization to avoid wire dislodgment.

d) Patients are seen by the team at 0630 A.M. Images, procedure, pathology report and consents are reviewed.

2.2 Surgery support:

Recommendation;

a) Patients are shifted to the operating room with admission note, pre-operative orders, consents, and site marking with patient's chart.

b) Patients are seen by the surgical team before shifting to the operating room to confirm the procedure, site marking, and reassurance to the patient.

c) Patients receive anxiolytic premedication such as lorazepam (valium), administered by anesthesia, to reduce patient anxiety before shifting to the operating room.

d) In the operating room, the patient is transferred carefully to the operating table in supine position with both arms at 90 degrees, and is secured. If the patient is scheduled *for reconstructive surgery, the plastic team should be available to direct their preferred positioning and preparation.*

e) *All needed forms such as pathology requests and labels are requested, printed, and filled completely and correctly before surgery is started.*

f) *If a para-vertebral nerve block or inter-pectoral block is considered by anesthesia, the patient is informed and consent obtained.*

g) *Bed sore prophylaxis and warmer blanket are applied when the patient is ready to sleep. If the patient is moderate-to-high risk for DVT, pneumatic stocking is applied when the patient is on the operating table and started when the patient is under anesthesia.*

h) *If the patient is going for sentinel lymph node biopsy, a hand-held gamma probe detector should be ready in the room and the breast pathology team should be informed before the procedure is started.*

i) *When an axillary procedure is planned, a shoulder gel pad should be applied under the scapula when the patient is intubated.*

j) *At the site of procedure, the chest wall from the neck and shoulder superiorly, upper abdomen inferiorly, medial half of other breast medially and lateral chest wall, axilla and upper arm laterally, are scrubbed with Povidon iodine paint.*

k) *If the sentinel lymph node is included in the procedure, it is preferred to start with that first and send it to pathology via the circulating nurse with a pathology request before approaching the breast.*

Note: *Do the exact procedure as indicated on the consent form. Any deviation during the procedure is rarely required, but if needed, the treating consultant should approach the family and discuss with them the intra-operative result and the needed procedures, and obtain a second consent from them on behalf of the patient.*

l) *After lumpectomy for breast cancer, the lumpectomy bed should be marked intra-operatively with clips to facilitate post-operative radiation therapy.*

m) Application of drain is part of the surgical procedure, and should be applied in the right place.

n) As part of post-operative pain control, it is preferable to apply local anesthesia (1% Lidocaine mixed with epinephrine) on wound edges before wound closure.

o) After the procedure is complete, the operative note and post-operative order checklist should be completed before the patient leaves the theater and prior to the next patient.

p) All surgical breast specimens (mastectomy or lumpectomy) should be marked with superior, inferior, lateral and medial margins and recorded on the pathology report.

q) Patient controlled anesthesia (PCA) is recommended as part of post-operative pain control in major surgeries such as bilateral breast mastectomy or bilateral reconstructive surgery.

2.3 Post-surgery support

Recommendation:

a) All patients are seen by the surgical team within 24 hours of the procedure (post-operative round checklist).

b) The surgical team discusses with the patient and their family the exact procedure, intraoperative findings, and answers any concerns.

c) Confirm that the patient is receiving an antibiotic, if needed; ambulating; pain free; using spirometer; seen by physiotherapy; and if they are ready for discharge.

3. Post-operative components:

The post-operative component begins at discharge and lasts until the patient is seen by the surgeon.

3.1 Discharge:

Recommendation:

a) All patients should receive their post-operative medications, discharge summary, and sick leave or work excuse.

b) The patient will be ready for discharge when oral intake is adequate, pain is controlled with analgesia, and she/he is capable of independent ambulation (usually on the first day after surgery).

c) All patients should receive an appointment in the surgical clinic after 2 weeks;, an appointment in the surgical wound clinic for wound and drain care, and for clips removal; and an appointment with the physiotherapy clinic (appointments checklist).

d) Post discharge order instructions should be clear for the wound care nurse regarding wound and drain care and for clips removal.

e) All patients are educated for wound and drain care by the assigned nurse.

f) Refer the patient to known providers of prostheses.

3.2 Post discharge support:

Recommendation:

a) The patients are seen in wound care clinic on day 3 after surgery for wound care, drain care and patient reassurance; the patient may take a shower before they come to the clinic.

b) Any concerns about the wound, daily wound care clinic appointments are needed.

c) On the 5th day after surgery, the patient is seen in wound nurse clinic for possible drain removal (drain care checklist).

d) The patient will be seen in physiotherapy clinic after removing the drain.

e) Three weeks post-surgery, the clips are removed in wound care clinic.

f) The patient will have appointments with wound care clinic until the drains and clips are removed and the wound is clean.

4 Follow-up care:

Recommendation:

a) *All patients will have follow-up with surgical clinic two weeks post-operatively to check the wound and discuss post-operative plan for adjuvant treatment.*

b) *Patients who underwent immediate breast reconstructive surgery have appointments with the plastic surgeon.*

c) *The patient is seen again in surgical clinic after three to six months.*

d) *After 6 months, patients with clean, healed wounds who are confirmed to have an appointment with an oncologist are discharged from surgical clinic, which will refer the patient back if any further surgery is needed in future.*

e) *Patients who underwent axillary surgery are followed by physiotherapy for shoulder.*

CLINCAL PATHWAY ON SPECIAL POPULATIONS;

PREGNANCY:

Risk of breast diseases in pregnant similar as non-pregnant patient, but be careful regarding staging with images, teratogenic effect of chemotherapy, other medicine and radiation treatment.

Recommendation:

a) Pregnant patients should have their pregnancy documented on the file in weeks of gestation.

b) It is preferred to add a colored sticker on the patient file to indicate that she is pregnant.

c) A pregnant patient should be provided with written information about her surgery and the risk of abortion/pre-term labor during or after the procedure, and sign the consent about that.

d) Pregnant patients should not receive any radiation during pregnancy to avoid child birth defects.

e) No images can be taken during pregnancy other than liver U/S and chest X-ray, with protective shields on her pregnant uterus.

f) Chemotherapy is safe during second and third trimester only; teratogenic effect is very high in the first trimester.

g) All patients should be seen by obstetrician before and after the surgery to assess the fetus and mother's condition.

h) Sentinel lymph node biopsy is still controversial for use in pregnant patients.

i) Avoid using any teratogenic medications and consult a clinical pharmacologist before giving any medications.

j) Avoid direct pressure on her abdomen procedure by surgeon and the assistants during breast surgery.

k) Opioid-free analgesia is preferred after surgery to avoid fetal effects.

l) Reconstructive surgery is prohibited during pregnancy because of breast engorgement and discrimination between both breasts

HIGH RISK:

High risk patients are who has High risk of mortality or morbidity during or after surgery, particularly with regard to organ failure, compared with other groups at lower risk. Most useful scoring system in surgical risk assessment remain the ASA score.

Recommendation;

a) All patients who been categorized as high risk should be admitted about 2 days before surgery to be assessed by consultant anesthesia and sub specialty as needed.

b) If the patient has any risk for surgery and need ICU bed or further investigation, anesthesiologist in pre anesthesia clinic should contact the treating surgical team and document the ASA of the patient and all needed investigations.

c) If ICU bed is required by anesthesia or breast surgical team, critical care unite should be contacted one week before the surgery to arrange ICU bed postoperatively.

d) high risk consent should be written on details and titled with HIGH RISK CONSENT on the file including patient full name, her/his disease, requested surgery and alternatives, risk of death or organ failure during or after anesthesia, and the patient and two witnesses are needed to sign the consent with their ID card number.

e) Patient refuse the treatment with high risk consent or refuse to sign the consent need to be documented in the file on details by treating team.

f) Renal failure cases (ESRD) need to do dialysis one day before the surgery.

EMERGENCY SURGERY

Emergency surgery is rarely indicated in breast as most of cases are cancer for neoplastic surgery or benign for waiting list. Most common emergency surgeries done in breast unit are breast abscess drainage or hematoma evacuation after mastectomy.

Recommendations

a) Full investigations including CBC, coagulation profile are needed before surgery

b) Prophylactic antibiotic is started as soon as the patient decided for surgery.

c) Notify theater and the on call anesthesiologist and complete an emergency form.

d) Treating team and on call team should be aware about the patient condition.

e) Any emergency cases done should be reported in the daily morning meeting next day.

OUTSIDE RESIDENTS

Recommendation;

a) Inform the patient before the first visit to Breast surgery clinic to bring all their images, medical reports, pathology slides and to stop aspirin if a biopsy was planned.

b) Arrange hospital accommodation and transportation by patient relations.

c) Inform the Patient to remain nearby after surgery for duration of 48 hours after discharge.

SURGICAL COMPLICATIONS

A variety of complications can occur in association with diagnostic and multidisciplinary Management procedures. Some of these complications are related to the breast itself, and others are associated with Axillary staging Procedures.

1. Hematoma and bleeding

Recommendation;

a) *Any hematological disease should be identified and treated before surgery*

b) *Stop the NSAID as aspirin and Plavix 10 days before the procedure.*

c) *Avoid using heparin and Low Molecular Weight Heparin (LMWH) as anti-thromboembolic prophylaxis, instead use stocking and intraoperative pneumatic cuff.*

d) *A high risk patient for bleeding should be referred to anti thrombotic team to have clear plane for tissue biopsy and surgery.*

e) *Proper homeostasis should be achieved during the surgery.*

f) *Pressure dressing in OR applied after covering the wound which can be removed after 24-48 hours.*

g) *6) Any patient who diagnosed with hematoma/bleeding, coagulation profile and hemoglobin level should be measured, 2 units of PRBC should be prepared, correct any coagulopathy, and prepare the patient for re-exploration and homeostasis.*

2. Wound infections and skin necrosis.

Recommendation

a) Give prophylactic antibiotics about 30 minutes before incision and if the procedure took longer than 4 hours, a second dose of antibiotic is recommend.

b) Post-operative antibiotics should be given to implant/tissue expander, diabetic, Neoadjuvant chemotherapy or wound complicated by hematoma.

c) Instruct the patient to stop smoking 2 months before procedure.

d) Avoid thin flaps to prevent flap necrosis and thick flaps to prevent cancer local recurrence

e) Control blood sugar in diabetic patients with sliding scale.

f) Instruct to reduce body weight before surgery

g) Avoid any unnecessarily blood transfusion

h) Personal hygiene is important before and after surgery.

i) If infection is diagnosed, open the wound to drain the collection, take a wound swab for culture and sensitivity, and start broad spectrum antibiotics with daily dressing as outpatient in the wound care nurse clinic, if the patient needs IV antibiotics, admission is arranged.

3. Seroma

Seroma is a collection of serous fluid in the dead space of the axilla and breast.

Recommendation

a) *Avoid premature removal of the drains.*
b) *Avoid aspiration of the Seroma because it will be absorbed after a few weeks, unless it is moderate to severe.*
c) *Patients with a Seroma do not need antibiotics unless the patient is diabetic, and obese.*
d) *4) Frequent follow-up is needed in surgical clinic and wound care nurse clinic until the Seroma is resolved.*

4. Chronic pain

Small number of patients who undergo breast surgery will experience chronic pain for several months, and the etiology is unknown but it is neuropathic in origin.

Analgesic and long-term follow-up is recommended until her pain is resolved and further opinion can be taken from pain control team.

5. Deep venous thrombosis (DVT)

Cancer is one of the risk factors for DVT, and prophylaxis should be taken with early mobilization and stocking.

Recommendations

a) *Patients who are on pharmacological antithrombotic agents for previous DVT or high risk for DVT, thromboembolic team should be involved with clear plan to avoid DVT or bleeding.*

b) *All patients should be inspected for sign of DVT.*

c) *Patients who develop DVT/PE, antithrombotic team and pulmonary team should be involved and apply direct pressure on mastectomy site to avoid hematoma formation when anticoagulant is started with close observation by assigned nurse, and treating team.*

Clinical Responsibilities of Residents and Specialists In breast surgery unit

❖ Resident

1) Junior

- Attend the Clinics with the Consultant / Specialist (refer to table page 25)
- Responsible for admissions, pre-operative orders, site marking and consent.
- Attend surgical Grand Round and Breast Tumor conference.
- On call team should attend the daily morning report.
- Attend pre-operative team round at 06:30 AM and post-operative team round after the last case of surgery with consultant, Specialist and senior resident.
- Be in OR at 07:15 AM and attend the surgery of all cases.
- Responsible to write post-operative orders, progress note, discharge note, post discharge orders, appointments, medications, accommodations, travel tickets, sick leave / work leave.

2) Senior

- Attend the Combined breast Clinic and complete the combined clinic form; (page 68), dictate medical report and place workup orders.
- Perform the procedures in the clinic as biopsy / Seroma aspiration / wound care with Specialist supervision and document it in the file.
- Attend the breast surgery clinic with the Consultant / Specialist (refer to table at the end of this document)

- For any issue in the clinic / OR /ward the senior Resident should inform the Specialist.
- Organize next week admissions for surgery with the Specialist.
- Contact the Plastic Surgery team if the patient is for reconstruction.
- Book the patients for sentinel, wire localization, ICU / overnight recovery, one week before the date of surgery.
- Refer the patients to other subspecialties.
- on call team should attend the daily morning report at 7; 30am.
- Supervise the duties of the Junior Resident.
- Confirm patients are booked for sentinel injection, wire localization, and the availability of ICU / overnight recovery on the morning of surgery.
- The Pathology report is the responsibility of the senior resident to be completed correctly and printed in OR.
- Attend all OR cases on the list at 07:30 AM.
- Operative note and post-operative orders should be documented in the file of the patient.
- Confirm discharge note, post discharge orders, appointments, drain care, wound care, medications, accommodations, sick leave / work leave are complete correctly with junior resident.
- Attend team round with the Consultant and Specialist at 06:30 AM.
- Attend surgical grand rounds and breast tumor conference.
- Complete Tumor Board conference forms (operative cases; page 69) after each operated case in OR and reviews them with Specialist before submitting them to secretary .

- The operated cases in breast tumor conference should be presented by the senior resident.

❖ Specialist

- Attend the combined Breast Clinic and complete the combined breast clinic; page 70, dictate the combined clinic medical report for each case seen and place workup orders.
- Responsible to attend the breast surgical clinics and confirm that all patients are Seen by the end of the clinic with the nurse including the charts review and no-show patients and reschedule them according to their priority.
- Confirm that the patients who are scheduled for OR and pre-anesthesia clinic are done correctly.
- Supervise the procedures done in the clinics by the Senior Residents as biopsy / Seroma aspiration / wound care.
- Arrange all the cases for next week surgery with the Consultant and with scheduling team .
- On call team should attend the daily morning report.
- Confirm the cases for next week admissions for surgery with the case manager, review them and confirm their date of admission, type of procedures and needed orders and discuss the plan with the Senior / Junior Residents (Plastic Surgeon, sentinel, wire localization, ICU / overnight, referral).
- Confirm patient's admission in the ward, the admission notes and preoperative Orders and consents are completed correctly by senior/junior resident.
- Confirm patients are scheduled for sentinel injections, wire localization, and the availability of ICU / overnight recovery with the Senior Resident.

- Lead the team round at 06:30 AM on day of surgery and after the last operated case with Senior / Junior Resident (knows the details of the cases, their procedures, and completeness of the orders and checklists).
- Confirm running of the OR cases on right time, and be available in theater at 07:15 AM for sign in, patient intubation and extubation, patient positioning, patient safety, correct procedure, and correct site marking, confirm to start the case with anesthesia.
- Contact plastic surgery team on the day of surgery
- Confirm the pathology reports are completed correctly in OR by senior resident.
- Confirm the breast tumor conference forms (operative cases) are completed correctly by the Senior Resident and submitted to secretary.
- Responsible to answer the residents questions, concerns and confirm their training progress in the unit.
- Responsible for dictation of medical reports, operative notes, and review the Resident's dictation of admission, discharge and sick leave / work leave.
- Confirm that all the patients are discharged with appointments, medications, accommodations, drain care, wound care are complete, and any delay for patient discharge should be discussed with the assigned nurse for that delay.
- Attend the surgical grand round and breast Tumor conference.
- Supervise the Senior Resident presentations for the operative cases in tumor board meeting.
- Confirm the patient's clinical pathway is running smoothly and on the right time.

Week schedule for breast surgery team unit

Day/time	06:30AM-07:15AM	07:30AM-08:30AM	08:30AM – 12:00 PM		1:00 PM - 5:00 PM	
Sunday	Team Round	Daily Morning Report 7:30-8:00	Operation / Post-operative team round			SAMPLE WEEKLY SCHEDULE OF BREAST SURGERY UNIT
			Combined breast clinic			
Monday			Operation / Post-operative team round			
Tuesday			Clinic		Call for next week cases	
					Operative cases for tumor board and research forms completed and submitted to secretary	
Wednesday			Review next week cases and orders / Breast team meeting		Clinic	
			Booking for sentinel / Wire localization/IORT*			
Thursday		Surgical Grand Round	Breast Tumor conference 08:30-10:00	Team round & Journal club 11:00-12:00	Endorsement for weekend team on call	
			Scheduling for surgery		ICU Bed Booking	

*IORT intraoperative radiotherapy.
Weekly schedule dependent on geographic location

Breast surgery clinical pathway

DOCTOR AND PATIENT RELATION AND CONFIDENTIALITY

- Each patient has the right to have full disclosure of the procedure and/or treatment and/or medication involved, and the right to agree or disagree with the procedure, treatment, or medication.

- Each patient's decision must be respected by the medical team, staff and administration without negative responses from any hospital personnel.

- Each patient must be respected should she or he later elect not to undergo the procedure, even if consent was given at an earlier time.

- The patient has the right to get the advice of outside counsel for a second opinion, without pressure or negative responses from the treating surgeon or any medical staff.

- Patients must not be forced into making hurried decisions for any purpose or reason. Each decision must be made with clear knowledge of all the facts.

- The patient has the right to be treated with equality and integrity regardless of social standing, income level or circumstance.

- Each patient should be given the same personal respect and treatment prior to, during and after any procedure or treatment.

- Doctors should not withhold information from the patient which may impact the patient's decision-making process.

- The doctor must disclose any experimental, unproven, trial or new procedures, treatments or medications, and equally advise the patient on potential outcomes or side effects, as well as benefits.

- Doctors and nursing staff must treat each patient with respect and dignity at all times, as patients may be experiencing varying levels of stress and concern which can affect their behavior and/or personality.

Breast surgery clinical pathway

- Patient details, circumstances or situations must only be discussed in regard to the patient's wellbeing or advancement of surgical or medical skill, and not subject for social forums or media exchanges.

UNDERGRADUATE AND POSTGRADUATE TRAINING

In the breast surgery unit, undergraduate medical students have frequent sessions, bed side teaching, and opportunities to attend the operation and present the clinic with breast surgical team, and participate in many teaching sessions at our institution.

Post graduate doctors and Specialists are part of the breast surgery team. They are involved in the breast surgery clinic, tumor board meeting, decision making, admission, and surgery, and their responsibilities are considered an integral part of breast surgery unit.

CHECKLISTS

Breast Diseases History

- ❖ Greet the patient
- ❖ Introduce yourself
- ❖ Confirm patient's identity
- ❖ Take permission

  - **Personal history**
    - Chief Complaint in Detail
    - Detailed History
    - Other Presenting Symptoms
      - *breast mass*
      - *breast erythema*
      - *breast pain*
      - *nipple discharge*
      - *nipple or skin retraction*
      - *axillary mass or pain*
      - *arm swelling*
      - *symptoms of metastatic spread (soft tissue, lung, bone, liver)*
    - Risk Factors for Breast Cancer
  - **Past Medical History of Breast Disease in Detail Family History of Breast and Other Cancers with Emphasis on Gynecological Cancers**
  - **Reproductive History**
    - *pregnant*
    - *age at menarche*
    - *age at first delivery*
    - *number of pregnancies, children and miscarriages*
    - *age at onset of menopause history of hormonal use including contraceptive pills and hormonal replacement therapy (type and duration)*
  - **Past Medical History**
  - **Past Surgical History**
  - **Medication History**

- ❖ Summarize the key findings and document
- ❖ Thank the patient

Breast surgery clinical pathway

Breast Physical Examination

- ❖ Vital Statistics
- ❖ Local Examination (Right, Left, Bilateral)

    Breast

    - Lump
        - *size*
        - *location*
        - *fixed to chest wall or fixed to skin*
        - *number of lumps*
    - Skin Changes
        - *erythema (localized, generalized)*
        - *edema (localized, generalized)*
        - *dimpling*
        - *infiltration*
        - *ulceration*
        - *satellite nodules*
        - *previous surgery scar*
    - Nipple and Areola Changes
        - *retraction*
        - *erythema*
        - *erosion and ulceration*
        - *discharge (bloody, green, serous ,milk)*

    Axilla

    - Lymphadenopathy
    - Lymph nodes are mobile or fixed
    - Palpable supra/infra clavicular and cervical LN

- ❖ General examination
- ❖ TNM
- ❖ Summarize your findings and document

COMBINED BREAST CLINIC ORDERS

- Complete blood count with differential (CBCD), coagulation profile, renal and hepatic profile.
- Pregnancy test if the patient is of child bearing age.
- Bilateral mammography and/or ultrasound.
- Chest x-ray or computed tomography imaging (CT) of the chest, if needed.
- Abdominal ultrasound or CT of the abdomen, if needed.
- Bone scan, if indicated.
- If the patient has neurological symptoms, CT/MRI brain is indicated.
- Electrocardiogram (ECG) and echocardiogram if the patient is going for chemotherapy, or has long standing high blood pressure, heart disease, or cardiac symptoms.
- MRI breast if lumpectomy (BCT) was planned.
- Core biopsy in the clinic if the lump is palpable or image-guided biopsy.
- Pre-anesthesia clinic if surgery is planned within two weeks.

PREOPERATIVE BREAST SURGERY ORDERS

- Complete blood count with differential (CBCD), and renal and hepatic profile.
- Coagulation profile (PT, PTT.INR).
- Chest x-ray, electrocardiogram (ECG).
- NPO at 12:00 midnight.
- Surgical consent.
- Site marking of surgery.
- Antibiotic prophylaxis IV, single dose at call for surgery.
    - Keflex 1g IV 30 minutes before incision (if patient's BMI >30, give 2g IV).
    - In penicillin allergy, Clarithromycin 600 mg IV 30 minutes before surgery.
- Deep venous thrombosis prophylaxis with graduated compression thromboembolic deterrent stockings (TEDs).

Orders for Sentinel Lymph Node Biopsy

- Check the request in ICIS under sentinel lymph node biopsy.
- Confirm booking of the patient for injection with nuclear medicine.
- If the patient is scheduled in OR as the first case, injection for sentinel should be done at 4:30 P.M. the day before surgery. If the patient is scheduled as the 2nd or 3rd case, sentinel should be done at 7:30 A.M. the day of surgery.
- Call the nuclear medicine department one day before surgery to confirm booking.
- Patient should be consented for radioisotope material injection.
- Site marking of injection.

Orders for Wire Localization

- Check the request in the ICIS under wire localization with image guided biopsy.
- Confirm the patient's booking with radiology.
- Schedule the patient for OR as 2nd or 3rd case to avoid OR delay.
- Call the radiology department one day before surgery.
- Patient should be consented for localization.
- Site marking of localization.

Operative Note Checklist

1) Date and time of surgery.

2) Name of consultant.

3) Name of the surgeon.

4) Name of assistants.

5) Name of anesthesiologist.

6) Type of anesthesia (GA, Local, Spinal, Sedation, etc.).

7) Pre-operative diagnosis.

8) Post-operative diagnosis.

9) Type and side of the surgery.

10) Clinical history.
    - brief history, and physical examination,
    - final diagnosis,
    - TNM,
    - Neoadjuvant treatment
    - clinical/radiological response

11) Procedure in detail, including:
    - Positioning,
    - type and site of incision,
    - intraoperative findings,
    - amount of bleeding,
    - the procedure done,
    - type of specimens removed (mastectomy, lumpectomy, etc.) and markings,
    - homeostasis, wound closure and dressing, and sentinel result,
    - type of reconstruction (implant or tissue expander),
    - name of plastic surgeon,
    - type, number and sites of the drains applied,
    - patient and wound condition after extubation,
    - *patient shifted to recovery room, then to ward or to ICU,*

POST OPERATIVE INSTRUCTIONS

A) Post-Operative Instructions for Mastectomy
B) Post-Operative Instructions for skin sparing Mastectomy
C) Post-Operative Instructions for Lumpectomy

A) Post-Operative Instructions for Mastectomy

- NPO until full recovery.
- IV fluid according to IV fluid protocol.
- Soft diet can be started 8 hours after surgery, if the patient tolerates it. D/C IV fluids, and start normal diet the next morning.
- Diabetic diet for diabetic patients and low salt diet for hypertensive patients.
- Anti-emetic such as metoclopramide 40 mg IV OD for 24 hours, then PRN.
- Pain control
  - Acetaminophen 1 g Q8hr IV for first 24 hours then PRN
  - After 24 hours, acetaminophen 1 gm P.O QID for 5 days
  - Opiates, including codeine preparations, tramadol, or morphine, should be reserved for severe pain. Whenever opiates are used, attention should be paid to prevent nausea and vomiting, and non-ambulation.
- If the patient was on PCA, stop it 24 hours after surgery and give acetaminophen 1 g QID IV for next 24 hours then PRN. After 24 hours, give acetaminophen 1 gm P.O QID for 5 days.
- Post-operative antibiotic according to the patient's risk of infection.
- Wound drain care (amount, color) and remove any other tubes such as NGT and Foley catheter.
- Remove the pressure dressing 24 hours after surgery.
- Change the dressing if it is soaked.
- Spirometry as soon as patient is awake (10 times/hr. for 3 days post-op) to avoid atelectasis.
- Encourage full mobilization out of the bed as soon as patient is awake.
  - Patient should be helped to chair by evening the day of surgery. This will be followed by gentle assisted mobilization inside and outside the room that evening or the next day to avoid DVT.

Breast surgery clinical pathway

- - If the patient is unable to move for medical reasons, encourage them to move their feet on bed with the help of the sitter.
- Physiotherapy referral.
- If the patient is diabetic, follow the diabetic patient protocol.
- If the patient was on anti-thrombotic treatment pre-op, there should be close monitoring and observation for any sign of bleeding. Follow anti thrombotic protocol and keep pressure dressing for 48 hours.
- Resume all pre-op medications post-operative, except anti thrombotic treatment (aspirin, Plavix, Warfarin, heparin).

B) Post-Operative Instructions for Skin Sparing Mastectomy

- NPO until full recovery and IV fluid according to the IV fluid protocol.
- Soft diet can be started 8-10 hours after surgery, if the patient tolerates it. D/C IV fluids, and start normal diet the next morning.
- Diabetic diet for diabetic patients and low salt diet for hypertensive patients.
- Anti-emetic such as metoclopramide 40mg IV OD for 24 hours, then PRN.
- Pain control
  - Acetaminophen 1g Q8hr IV for first 24 hours, then PRN
  - After 24 hours, acetaminophen 1gm P.O QID for 5 days
  - Opiates, including codeine preparations, tramadol, or morphine should be reserved for severe pain. Whenever opiates are used, attention should be paid to prevent nausea, and vomiting.
- PCA is indicated in bilateral breast surgery and should be requested by anesthesiologist in OR.
- If the patient was on PCA, stop it 24 hours after surgery and give acetaminophen 1g QID IV for next 24 hours, then PRN. After 24 hours, give acetaminophen 1gm P.O QID for 5 days.
- Post-operative antibiotic for 5 days.
- Wound drain care: (note amount, color) and remove any other tubes as NGT and Foley catheter.
- Wound assessment and dressing with plastic team.
- Change the dressing if it is soaked.
- Spirometry as soon as patient is awake (10 times /hr. for 3 days post-op) to avoid atelectasis.
- Encourage full mobilization out of the bed as soon as patient is awake.
  - Patient should be helped to a chair by evening of the day of surgery. This will be followed by gentle assisted mobilization inside and outside the room that evening or the next day to avoid DVT.
  - If the patient is unable to move for medical reasons, encourage them to move their feet on the bed with the help of the sitter.
- If the patient is diabetic, follow the diabetic patient protocol.
- If the patient was on anti-thrombotic treatment pre-op, there should be close monitoring and observation for any sign of bleeding. Follow anti thrombotic protocol and keep pressure dressing for 48 hours.
- Resume all pre-op medications post-operative, except anti thrombotic treatment (aspirin, Plavix, Warfarin, heparin)

C) **Post-Operative Instructions for Lumpectomy**

- NPO until full recovery and IV fluid according to the IV fluid protocol.
- Soft diet can be started 8-10 hours after surgery, if the patient tolerates it. D/C IV fluid and start normal diet the next morning.
- Diabetic diet for diabetic patients and low salt diet for hypertensive patients.
- Anti-emetic such as metoclopramide 10mg IV BID for 24 hours, then PRN.
- Pain control
    - Acetaminophen 1g BID IV for 24 hours
    - After 24 hours, acetaminophen 1 gm P.O QID for 5 days.
    - Opiates, including codeine preparations, Tramadol, or morphine, should be reserved for severe pain. Whenever opiates are used, attention should be paid to prevent nausea and vomiting.
- Post-operative antibiotic according to the patient's risk of infection.
- Patients should begin wearing sponge bra as an extra pressure on the breast to prevent fluid collection as soon as they arrive on ward.
- Remove any tubes such as NGT and Foley catheter.
- Remove the pressure dressing 24 - 48 hours after surgery.
- Change the dressing if it is soaked.
- Spirometry as soon as patient is awake (10 times/hr. for 3 days post-op) to avoid atelectasis.
- Encourage mobilization out of the bed as soon as patient is awake.
    - Patient should be helped to a chair by evening of the day of surgery, followed by gentle assisted mobilization inside and outside the room that evening or next day to avoid DVT.
    - If the patient is unable to move for medical reasons, encourage them to move their feet on the bed with the help of the sitter.
- If the patient is diabetic, follow the diabetic patient protocol.
- If the patient was on anti-thrombotic treatment pre-op, there should be close monitoring and observation for any sign of bleeding, and follow anti thrombotic protocol.
- Resume all pre-op medications post-operative, except anti thrombotic treatment (aspirin, Plavix, Warfarin, and Heparin).

WHEN TO CALL THE RESIDENT

- If there is any sign of accumulation of blood (hematoma) on chest wall and/or axilla, such as swelling, continuous bleeding through the drain or dropping of hemoglobin.
- High grade fever >38°C post-operatively.
- Tachypnea, tachycardia, hypotension or chest pain.

Summary of Mastectomy /axillary dissection orders

Preoperative orders in clinic

Type of surgery;

- Simple mastectomy
- Modified radical mastectomy
- Mastectomy with sentinel lymph node biopsy

Admission order;

- Pre anesthesia new follow-up
- Pre anesthesia walk in new follow-up (if surgery within 2 weeks)
- Pre anesthesia follow-up (if seen before by anesthesia)
- Admit to surgery breast /Endo

Investigations;

- Complete blood count (CBC)
- Coagulation profile PT, PTT, INR
- Hepatitis screening (hepatitis C antibody, hepatitis B S antigen, hepatitis B, S antibody)
- UCG, Urine (child bearing age female)
- Renal profile
- ECG
- Blood glucose if diabetic
- Chest x ray AP/Lateral if no CT scan done
- Echocardiogram +/-stress test (long standing hypertension>10 years, cardiac disease symptoms, history of cardiac disease)

Consultation (complete consultation form);

- Nephrology (renal impairment or ESRD)
- Cardiology (cardiac disease symptoms, history of cardiac disease, ECG changes, abnormal echocardiogram)
- Pulmonary (respiratory disease, on methotrexate medications)
- Anticoagulant team (heparin, warfarin, claxan, LMWH)

Book for overnight recovery /ICU if;

- Cardiac problem /ICU admission
- Respiratory failure
- Overweight, BMI >40
- Recommended by anesthesia

Breast surgery clinical pathway

Patient advice before surgery;

- Stop following medications 10 days before surgery; Aspirin, Plavix
- Control blood sugar, high blood pressure, bronchial asthma (primary health care physician at local hospital)
- Reduce weight BMI >30
- Stop smoking at least 10 days before surgery
- take shower day of admission

Preoperative orders in surgical ward
- Vital signs at arrival

Investigations;

- CBC if more than 1 month
- Coagulation profile (PT, PTT, INR) if more than one month or patient on anticoagulant medications)
- Blood glucose level
- Diabetic (high blood sugar sliding scale protocol)

Consultations

- Anticoagulation team (heparin, warfarin, LMWH, DVT/PE)
- OB/GY in pregnant
- Cardiology if not seen in Outpatient

Surgery preparation;

- NPO at 12 MN
- IV Fluid Dextrose 5% 0.45% NaCl 35cc/Kg (**except** renal and cardiac patients follow nephron/cardiac IVF protocol)
- Shave axilla at morning 5; 00am
- Shower with both breasts and axilla cleaning with antiseptic soap/lotion at 6; 00am,
- Do not put on any lotion, cream, powder, makeup or perfume on neck.
- Evacuate bladder when call for surgery
- Take regular medications with sips of water (hypertensive medications, thyroid medications)
- Site marking
- Surgical Consent
- Sentinel lymph node injection in nuclear medicine department (as ordered in clinic)
- Remove all Metal objects. Remove all jewelry, including <u>all</u> body piercings
- before taken into the operating room, remove eyeglasses, hearing aid(s), dentures, prosthetic device(s), and scarf.

Breast surgery clinical pathway

- Gown, head and shoe cover and stocking
- Remove contact lenses, hair clips, accessories, nail polish and underwear, if patient is menstruating, use disposable or cotton underwear.
- Antibiotic prophylaxis IV, single dose at call for surgery, Keflex 1g IV 30 minutes before incision, if patient BMI >30 give 2 g IV.
- In penicillin allergy, clarithromycin 600 mg IV 30 minutes before surgery.
- Deep venous thrombosis prophylaxis with graduated compression thromboembolic deterrent stockings (TEDs).

Post-operative order

Day 0 (surgery day)
- Vital signs q 1 hour for 4 hours (arrive from operating room)
- Vital signs q 4 hours for 24 hours

IV fluid
- IV Fluid Dextrose 5% 0.45% NaCl 35 cc/Kg (**except** renal and cardiac patients follow nephrology/cardiac IVF protocol)

Dietary
- NPO until full recovery 8 hours after patient arrive to surgical ward
- Sips of water after 8 hours
- Stop IVF if oral fluid is tolerated
- Soft diet if patient tolerate oral fluid

Consultation
- OB/GY in pregnant

Medication
- Acetaminophen 1 g IV q 6 hour for 24 hours, in case of Bilateral breast surgery; PCA is indicated for 24 hours
- Acetaminophen –codeine **(300mg-30mg)** tab PRN
- Metoclopramide 20 mg IV BID for 24 hours
- Keflex 500 mg Oral Q6 hr for 10 days.
- Don't start aspirin, anticoagulation, Plavix (doctor instruction)

Wound care;

- Check wound q1 hour for 4 hours then q4 hour for 24 hours
- Change the wound dressing if heavy soaked with blood (notify MD)

Drain care;

- Measure output q 12 hours
- Observe for drain fluid color

Physical therapy

- Spirometer training 10 times per hour
- Mobilization outside the bed

Day 1 (24 hours post-operative)
- Vital signs q 6-8 hours for 24 hours

Dietary

- Normal diet

Medication

- Acetaminophen 1 gm **IV** PRN
- Acetaminophen 1 g **PO** q 6 hour for 5 days
- Acetaminophen –codeine **(300mg-30mg)** tab PRN
- Metoclopramide 20 mg **IV** PRN
- Regular chronic disease medications
- Continue on cancer therapy (e.g. famara, Herceptin, tamoxifen)
- don't start aspirin, anticoagulation, Plavix (doctor instruction)

Consultation

- Physiotherapy (sentinel lymph node, axillary lymph node dissection)

Wound care;

- Take shower
- Wound dressing

Physical therapy

- Spirometer training 10 times per hour
- Mobilization outside the room

Breast surgery clinical pathway

Discharge orders

All Patients are discharge after 24 hours of surgery
When to Discharge;

- Patient taking oral fluid
- No sign of hematoma or skin necrosis

Discharge Medications

- Acetaminophen 1 gm PO Q8 hours for 5 days
- Acetaminophen –codeine **(300mg-30mg)** tab PRN
- Oral Keflex 500 mg Q 6 hours for 10 days
- Chronic disease medications

Appointments;

- Wound care nurse clinic 48 hours after discharge for wound/drain care
- Wound care nurse clinic 3 weeks after discharge for clips removal
- Breast surgery clinic after 2 weeks
- Physiotherapy after 2 weeks

Immediate Notifying MD

- Persistent Bleeding/swelling (dressing is heavy soaked with blood)
- Persistent blood in drain
- Chest wall swelling (hematoma)

Summary of Skin sparing Mastectomy /axillary dissection orders

Preoperative orders in clinic

Type of surgery;

- Skin spring Mastectomy with sentinel lymph node biopsy
- Skin spring mastectomy with axillary dissection
- Skin spring mastectomy
- Tissue expander /implant insertion

Admission order;

- Pre anesthesia new follow-up
- Pre anesthesia walk in new follow-up (if surgery within 2 weeks)
- Pre anesthesia follow-up (if seen before by anesthesia)
- Admit to surgery breast /Endo

Investigations;

- Complete blood count (CBC)
- Coagulation profile PT, PTT, INR
- Hepatitis screening (hepatitis C antibody, hepatitis B S antigen, hepatitis B S antibody)
- UCG, Urine (child bearing age female)
- Renal profile
- ECG
- Blood glucose if diabetic
- Chest x ray AP/Lateral if no CT scan done
- Echocardiogram +/-stress test (long standing hypertension>10 years, cardiac disease symptoms, history of cardiac disease)

Consultation (complete consultation form)

- Plastic surgery
- Nephrology (renal impairment or ESRD)
- Cardiology (cardiac disease symptoms, history of cardiac disease, ECG changes, abnormal echocardiogram)
- Pulmonary (respiratory disease ,on methotrexate medications)
- Anticoagulant team (heparin, warfarin, claxan, LMWH)

Book for overnight recovery if;

- Cardiac problem /ICU admission
- Respiratory failure
- Overweight, BMI >40
- Recommended by anesthesia

Patient advice before surgery;

- Stop following medications 10 days before surgery; Aspirin, Plavix
- Control blood sugar, high blood pressure, bronchial asthma (primary health care physician at local hospital)
- Reduce weight BMI >30
- Stop smoking at least 10 days before surgery

Preoperative orders in surgical ward

- Vital signs at arrival

Investigations;

- CBC if more than 1 month
- Coagulation profile (PT, PTT, INR) if more than one month or patient on anticoagulant medications)
- Blood glucose level
- Diabetic (high blood sugar sliding scale protocol)

Consultations

- Anticoagulation team (heparin, warfarin, LMWH, DVT/PE)
- OB/GY in pregnant patient
- Cardiology if not seen in Outpatient
- Plastic surgery

Surgery preparation;

- NPO at 12 MN
- IV Fluid Dextrose 5% 0.45% NaCl 35cc/Kg (**except** renal and cardiac patients follow nephron/cardiac IVF protocol)
- Shave axilla at morning 5; 00am
- Shower with both breasts and axilla cleaning with antiseptic soap/lotion at 6; 00am,
- Do not put on any lotion, cream, powder, makeup or perfume on neck.
- Evacuate bladder when call for surgery

- Take regular medications with sips of water (hypertensive medications, thyroid medications)
- Site marking
- Surgical Consent
- Sentinel lymph node injection in nuclear medicine department (as ordered in clinic)
- Remove all Metal objects. Remove all jewelry, including <u>all</u> body piercings
- Before taken into the operating room, remove eyeglasses, hearing aid(s), dentures, prosthetic device(s), and scarf
- Gown, head and shoe cover and stocking
- Remove contact lenses, hair clips, accessories, nail polish and underwear, if patient is menstruating, use disposable or cotton underwear.
- Antibiotic prophylaxis IV, single dose at call for surgery, Keflex 1g IV 30 minutes before incision, if patient BMI >30 give 2 g IV.
- In penicillin allergy, clarithromycin 600 mg IV 30 minutes before surgery
- Deep venous thrombosis prophylaxis with graduated compression thromboembolic deterrent stockings (TEDs).

Post-operative order

Day 0 (surgery day)

- Vital signs q 1 hour for 4 hours (arrive from operating room)
- Vital signs q 4 hours for 24 hours

IV fluid

- IV Fluid Dextrose 5% 0.45% NaCl 35 cc/Kg (**except** renal and cardiac patients follow nephrology/cardiac IVF protocol)

Dietary

- NPO until full recovery 8 hours after patient arrive to surgical ward
- Sips of water after 8 hours
- Stop IVF if oral fluid is tolerated
- Soft diet if patient tolerate oral fluid

Consultation

- OB/GY in pregnant *patient*

Medication

- Acetaminophen 1 g IV q 6 hour for 24 hours, in case of Bilateral breast surgery; PCA is indicated for 24 hours
- Acetaminophen –codeine **(300mg-30mg)** tab PRN
- Metoclopramide 20 mg IV BID for 24 hours
- Keflex 500 mg Oral Q6 hr for 10 days.
- **<u>Don't start aspirin, anticoagulation, Plavix (doctor instruction)</u>**

Wound care;
- Check wound q1 hour for 4 hours then q4 hour for 24 hours
- Change the wound dressing if heavy soaked with blood (notify MD)

Drain care;

- Measure output q 12 hours
- Observe for fluid color

Physical therapy

- Spirometer training 10 times per hour
- Mobilization outside the bed

Day 1 (24 hours post-operative)
- Vital signs q 6 hours for 24 hours

Dietary

- Normal diet

Medication

- Acetaminophen 1 gm <u>IV</u> Q6hr for 24 hrs.
- Acetaminophen –codeine **(300mg-30mg)** tab PRN
- Metoclopramide 20 mg <u>IV</u> PRN
- Regular chronic disease medications
- Continue on cancer therapy (e.g. famara, Herceptin, tamoxifen)
- **<u>don't start aspirin, anticoagulation, Plavix (doctor instruction)</u>**

Consultation

- Physiotherapy (sentinel lymph node, axillary lymph node dissection)
- Plastic surgery review

Wound care;

- Take shower
- Wound dressing
- Supportive bra

Physical therapy

- Spirometer training 10 times per hour
- Mobilization outside the room

Immediate Notifying MD

- Persistent Bleeding/swelling (dressing is heavy soaked with blood)
- Persistent blood in drain (bleeding)

Discharge orders

All Patients are discharge after 48-72 hours of surgery.

When to Discharge;

- Plastic surgery approve for discharge
- Taking and tolerate oral fluid
- No sign of hematoma or skin necrosis

Discharge Medications

- Acetaminophen 1 gm PO Q6 hours for 5 days
- Acetaminophen –codeine **(300mg-30mg)** tab PRN
- Oral Keflex 500 mg Q 6 hours for 10 days
- Chronic disease medications

Appointments;

- Wound care nurse clinic 48 hours after discharge
- Breast surgery clinic after 2 weeks
- Physiotherapy after 2 weeks (axillary surgery)
- Plastic surgery appointment

Summary of Lumpectomy /axillary lymph node dissection orders

Preoperative orders in clinic

Type of surgery;

- Lumpectomy
- Lumpectomy with axillary dissection
- Lumpectomy with sentinel lymph node biopsy

Admission order;

- Pre anesthesia new follow-up
- Pre anesthesia walk in new follow-up (if surgery within 2 weeks)
- Pre anesthesia follow-up (if seen before by anesthesia)
- Admit to surgery breast /Endo

Investigations;

- Complete blood count (CBC)
- Coagulation profile PT, PTT, INR
- Hepatitis screening (hepatitis C antibody, hepatitis B S antigen, hepatitis B S antibody)
- UCG, Urine (child bearing age female)
- Renal profile
- ECG
- Blood glucose if diabetic
- Chest x ray AP/Lateral if no CT scan done
- Echocardiogram +/-stress test   (long standing hypertension>10 years, cardiac disease symptoms, history of cardiac disease)

Consultation (complete consultation form)

- Nephrology (renal impairment or ESRD)
- Cardiology (cardiac disease symptoms, history of cardiac disease, ECG changes, abnormal echocardiogram)
- Pulmonary (respiratory disease, on methotrexate medications)
- Anticoagulant team (heparin, warfarin, claxan, LMWH)

Book for overnight recovery /ICU if;

- Cardiac problem /ICU admission
- Respiratory failure
- Overweight, BMI >40
- Recommended by anesthesia

Patient advice before surgery;

- Stop following medications 10 days before surgery; Aspirin, Plavix
- Control blood sugar, high blood pressure, bronchial asthma (primary health care physician at local hospital)
- Reduce weight BMI >30
- Stop smoking at least 10 days before surgery

Preoperative orders in surgical ward

- Vital signs at arrival

Investigations;

- CBC if more than 1 month
- Coagulation profile (PT, PTT, INR) if more than one month or patient on anticoagulant medications)
- Blood glucose level
- Diabetic (high blood sugar sliding scale protocol)

Consultations

- Anticoagulation team (heparin, warfarin, LMWH, DVT/PE)
- OB/GY in pregnant
- Cardiology if not seen in Outpatient

Surgery preparation;

- NPO at 12 MN
- IV Fluid Dextrose 5% 0.45% NaCl 35cc/Kg (**except** renal and cardiac patients follow nephron/cardiac IVF protocol)
- Shave axilla at morning 5; 00am
- Shower with both breasts and axilla cleaning with antiseptic soap/lotion at 6; 00am,
- do not put on any lotion, cream, powder, makeup or perfume on neck.
- Evacuate bladder when call for surgery
- Take regular medications with sips of water (hypertensive medications, thyroid medications)
- Site marking
- Surgical Consent
- Sentinel lymph node injection in nuclear medicine department (as ordered in clinic)
- remove all Metal objects. Remove all jewelry, including <u>all</u> body piercings
- Before taken into the operating room, remove eyeglasses, hearing aid(s), dentures, prosthetic device(s), and scarf

Breast surgery clinical pathway

- Gown, head and shoe cover and stocking
- Remove contact lenses, hair clips, accessories, nail polish and underwear, if patient is menstruating, use disposable or cotton underwear.
- Antibiotic prophylaxis IV, single dose at call for surgery, Keflex 1g IV 30 minutes before incision, if patient BMI >30 give 2 g IV.
- In penicillin allergy, clarithromycin 600 mg IV 30 minutes before surgery.
- Deep venous thrombosis prophylaxis with graduated compression thromboembolic deterrent stockings (TEDs).

Post-operative order

Day 0 (surgery day)
- Vital signs q 1 hour for 4 hours (arrive from operating room)
- Vital signs q 4 hours for 24 hours

IV fluid
- IV Fluid Dextrose 5% 0.45% NaCl 35 cc/Kg (**except** renal and cardiac patients follow nephrology/cardiac IVF protocol)

Dietary
- NPO until full recovery 8 hours after patient arrive to surgical ward
- Sips of water after 8 hours
- Stop IVF if oral fluid is tolerated
- Soft diet if patient tolerate oral fluid

Consultation
- OB/GY in pregnant

Medication
- Acetaminophen 1 g IV q 6 hour for 24 hours.
- Acetaminophen –codeine **(300mg-30mg)** tab PRN
- Metoclopramide 20 mg IV BID for 24 hours
- Keflex 500 mg Oral Q6 hr for 5-10 days.
- **Don't start aspirin, anticoagulation, Plavix (doctor instruction)**

Wound care;
- Check wound q1 hour for 4 hours then q4 hour for 24 hours
- Change the wound dressing if heavy soaked with blood (notify MD)
- Supportive bra

Breast surgery clinical pathway

Drain care;

- Measure output q 12 hours
- Observe for drain fluid color

Physical therapy

- Spirometer training 10 times per hour
- Mobilization outside the bed then outside the room

Day 1 (24 hours post-operative)

- Vital signs q 6-8 hours for 24 hours

Dietary

- Normal diet

Medication

- Acetaminophen 1 gm **IV** PRN
- Acetaminophen 1 g **PO** q 6 hour for 5 days
- Acetaminophen –codeine **(300mg-30mg)** tab PRN
- Metoclopramide 20 mg **IV** PRN
- Regular chronic disease medications
- Continue on cancer therapy (e.g. famara, Herceptin, tamoxifen)
- **don't start aspirin, anticoagulation, Plavix (doctor instruction)**

Consultation

- Physiotherapy (sentinel lymph node, axillary lymph node dissection)

Wound care;

- Take shower
- Wound dressing

Physical therapy

- Spirometer training 10 times per hour
- Mobilization outside the room

Discharge orders

All Patients are discharge within 24 hours of surgery
When to Discharge;

- Patient taking oral fluid
- No sign of hematoma or bleeding

Discharge Medications

- Acetaminophen 1 gm PO Q8 hours for 5 days
- Acetaminophen –codeine **(300mg-30mg)** tab PRN
- Oral Keflex 500 mg Q 6 hours for 5 -10 days

Appointments;

- Wound care nurse clinic 48 hours after discharge for wound/drain care.
- Breast surgery clinic after 2 weeks
- Physiotherapy after 2 weeks (axillary surgery)

Immediate Notifying MD

- Persistent Bleeding/swelling (dressing is heavy soaked with blood)
- Persistent blood in drain

Daily Progress Note Checklist

1) Date and time of round

2) Name of consultant

3) Brief synopsis of patient condition, including surgery performed and how many days post-operative (for example, day 2 post right skin sparing mastectomy and axillary with tissue expander for multifocal breast cancer)

4) Ask the patient for any complaints (pain, dyspnea, chest pain, etc.)

5) Ask if oral fluids have been started and tolerated.

6) Describe general condition of the patient, including vital signs (fully awake, drowsy, semi-conscious, etc.)

7) Wound evaluation (sign of hematoma, infection, flap necrosis, bleeding, etc.)

8) Drain evaluation (amount and color).

9) Check upper and lower limbs for signs of DVT.

10) Encourage ambulation.

11) Give painkiller if patient is still complaining of pain

12) D/C IVF if oral fluid is tolerated.

13) Change dressing if it is soaked.

Drain Care Checklist

The drain care is started from the time of drain insertion in OR until the drain is removed in wound care nurse clinic.

1) Document the correct drain location on chest wall in operating room.

2) Observe for the amount and color of drainage, and exclude bleeding (persistent pure blood with or without clots in the bag).

3) Document the drain output (amount and color) in the patient chart daily as part the of progress note.

4) Absence of output indicates drain line blockage or kink. It can be treated by gentle manipulation at the drain site.

5) Keep the bag on negative pressure all the time. Failure to keep the bag on negative pressure should trigger assessment.

6) The drain line should be short and secured to the patient to avoid drain dislodgment during patient mobilization.

7) The drain bag should be easy to approach for evacuation or to assess color.

8) Regular assessment of drain site is important to monitor for bleeding and infection.

9) Clear instructions about drain care and how to evacuate, measure, and document the content on daily basis should be given to the patient and the supporter.

10) Drain is usually removed on the 5th day after surgery when output is less than 30ml and serous.

11) When drain removal is planned, explain the procedure to the patient. Drain site should be cleaned and covered. Document the date of removal of the drain.

BREAST TEAM ROUNDS

1. **PRE OPERATIVE BREAST TEAM ROUND (Day of surgery, 06:30 A.M.-07:15 A.M.)**
   - Check for Tumor Board Meeting management plan.
   - Check for breast surgery clinic note.
   - Examine the patient and confirm the correct procedure, correct side, and correct patient.
   - Check patient consent for breast/axilla procedure and for reconstructive procedure.
   - Review images and histopathology report.
   - Review pre-operative order.
   - Review if the patient is scheduled for sentinel LN biopsy and whether nuclear medicine has been contacted.
   - Review if the patient is scheduled for wire localization and whether radiology has been contacted.
   - Review if the patient took neoadjuvant chemotherapy, and if so, what was the last dose.

2. **POST OPERATIVE BREAST TEAM ROUND (end of the day of surgery and next morning)**

    - Explain to the patient the intraoperative findings and the procedure that has been done.

    - Confirm that the patient recovered from anesthesia with stable vital signs.

    - Check for any sign of bleeding/hematoma, skin necrosis at chest wall, sign of wound infection, or seroma.

    - Check drain site for any bleeding and check drain bag content (amount and color).

    - Check for pain control, and give analgesia if patient has pain.

    - Confirm the patient has started oral fluid and diet intake, and stop IV fluid.

    - Confirm if patient received antibiotics.

    - Examine both lower limbs for any sign of DVT (pain, swelling, redness). If there is, ultrasound of lower limb should be requested.

    - Encourage the patient to use the spirometer.

    - Confirm the patient resumes pre-operative medications for chronic diseases (diabetes, high blood pressure, seizure), except anti thrombotic medication, which can be restarted as the thromboembolic team recommends.

    - If the patient was in the ICU, patient should be cleared by the critical care doctor before discharge to the ward (patient is alert, cooperative, pain free, warm, normotensive, urine output >0.5 ml/kg/hr). Any central line should be removed, and a peripheral line is secured.

    - Explain to the patient about arm and shoulder exercise, and confirm the patient has physiotherapy appointment.

    - Confirm patient mobilization inside and outside the room.

    - Confirm if the patient is ready for discharge.

DISCHARGE CHECKLIST

Patients undergoing mastectomy or lumpectomy are ready to be discharged 24 hours after surgery, or 72 hours after surgery for patients undergoing reconstructive surgery.

- Patient is scheduled for follow up appointments
- Wound and drain care education
- Patient receives medications (painkiller, antibiotics, others)
- Patient receives a sick leave/work leave excuse
- Tickets and accommodation if patient is an outside resident
- Discharge summary
- Post discharge assessment for wound, drain and clips care to wound care nurse clinic.

APPOINTMENTS CHECKLIST

- Appointment with the treating surgeon two weeks post-discharge
- Appointment with the wound care nurse for wound and drain care the day after discharge, with post discharge orders
- Appointments with wound care nurse clinic five days post-discharge for possibility of drain removal
- Appointment with wound care nurse three weeks post-discharge for clips removal. If the patient is an outside resident, give clips removal form with clips removal device for removal of clips in her/ his province.
- Appointment with physiotherapy
- Appointment with thromboembolic team if patient is was on heparin or Warfarin, or if surgery was complicated by venous thromboembolic (DVT/PE)
- Appointment with subspecialty if patient was seen by other teams and needs further follow-up.

Post-Discharge Assessment for Wound Care Nurse

The wound and drain care starts the 2nd or 3rd day after discharge. Advise the patient to take shower before coming for wound dressing.

1 day post-discharge:

- Wound should be assessed for any signs of infection such as redness, tenderness, swelling, hotness or purulent discharge, or skin color changes (skin necrosis).
- Drain assessment for output color, and confirm patient knows how to evacuate, measure, and document the drainage.
- Wound dressing for breast surgery and drain with antiseptic and cover with dressing.

3 days post-discharge:

- Assess the wound for any signs of infection or skin necrosis, and complete dressing.
- Drain assessment for output color, and confirm patient knows how to evacuate, measure, and document the drainage.
- Wound dressing for breast surgery and drain with antiseptic and cover with dressing.

5 days post-discharge:

- Check for the wound for any sign of infection or Seroma formation
- Confirm drain output and met the criteria to remove the drain:
    1. Drain fluid is serous
    2. Drain output less than 30 ml in the last 24 hours
    3. No sign of seroma or infection.
- If it is decided to remove the drain, explain the procedure to the patient, and document removal of the drain on patient's file.
- If the drain is not removed at this time, give the patient another appointment to confirm drain removal.

3 weeks post-operative:

- Assess the wound for signs of infection, seroma
- Remove the wound clips and cover the wound line with steri-strips.

When to call the treating team
- Skin necrosis (dark red or black color of skin)
- Wound infection (redness, hotness, tenderness, swelling, purulent discharge)
- Seroma/hematoma (diffuse swelling, fluctuation)
- Drainage output is purulent

When to discharge from wound care nurse clinic;
- Wound is clean and healed
- No sign of infection, skin necrosis or Seroma
- Clips are removed
- Drain is removed

Wound Care Checklist

Wound care is started with skin care before, during and after surgery.

Skin Care Before Surgery

- Patient should shower with antiseptic solution or soap before coming to the hospital for admission and on the morning of surgery, and avoid putting powder, deodorant, perfume or cream on breast or axilla skin after showering.
- Axillary hair shaving on the morning of surgery should be done with clippers, not blade.

Skin Care During Surgery

- Skin should be handled carefully; avoid crushing the skin with instruments or burning it with diathermy.
- Homeostasis is a critical point for wound care.
- Wound should be closed in layers with subcutaneous tissue, then skin with clips, or cosmetic subcuticular closure after application of local anesthesia.

Skin Care After Surgery

- Wound of the breast and drain site are separately covered with proper dressing, and then covered with pressure dressing for 24 - 48 hours.
- For reconstructive surgery cases, the wound needs to be evaluated by the plastic surgery team on a daily basis.
- Drain site and the surface of pressure dressing should be assessed for bleeding before the patient leaves the operating room, recovery room, and the surgical ward.
- After 24-48 hours, the pressure dressing is removed and the wound is assessed for any sign of hematoma formation and flap necrosis, and then regular wound dressing is done.
- When discharge is planned, the patient can shower with the wound covered, avoiding any rubbing on the wound site. After shower, a regular dressing should be done before the patient is discharged to home.

Skin Care After Discharge

- The patient will have an appointment with Nurse Wound Care Clinic on the 3rd day after surgery for wound dressing.
- Patient can shower at home before she appears at Nurse Clinic for wound dressing.
  Wound should be observed for infection and seroma.

Breast surgery clinical pathway

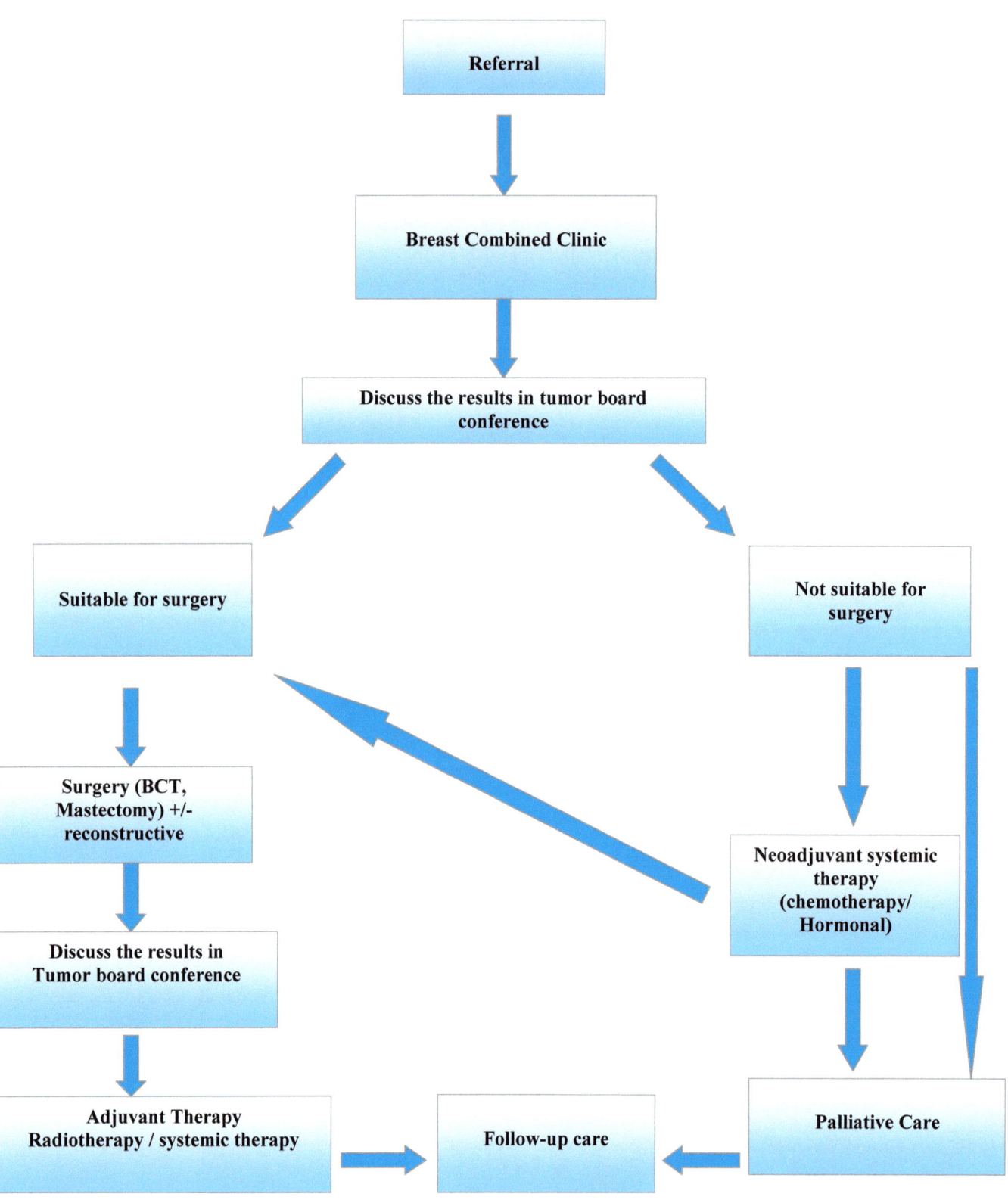

Figure 1. Breast cancer: The patient's pathway

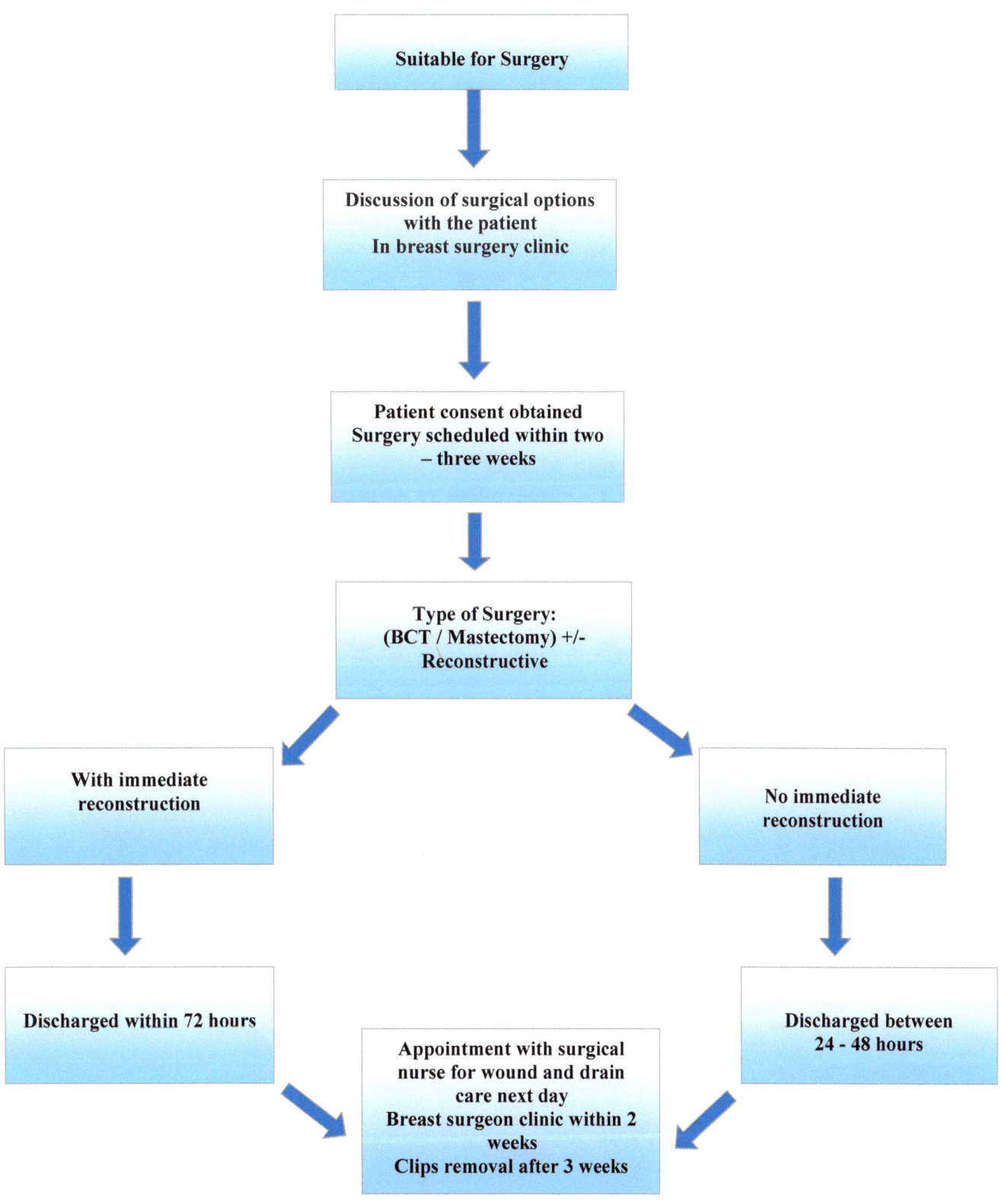

Figure 2. Surgical Treatment Journey

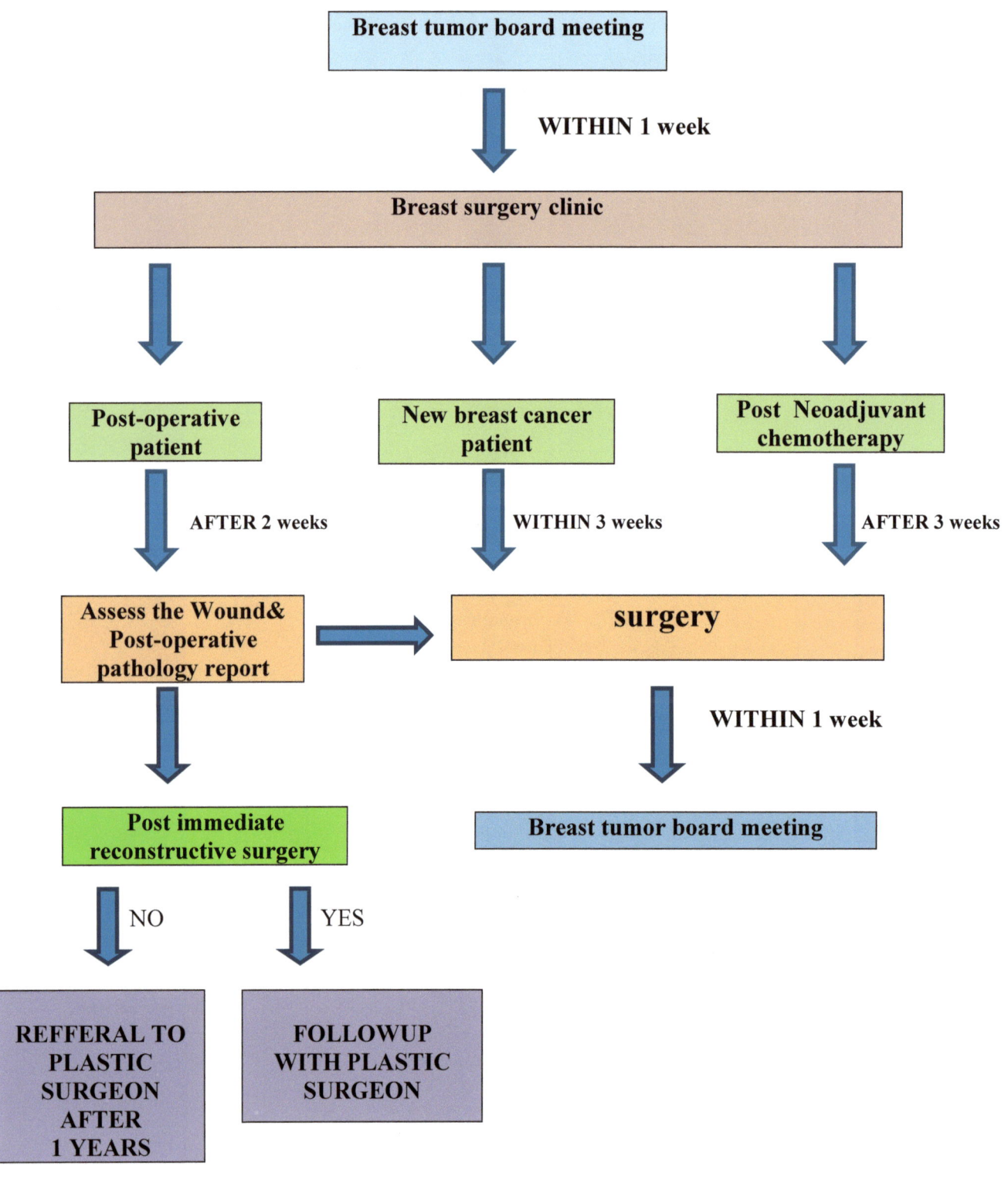

Figure 3. Patient's journey after breast tumor board meeting

BREAST TUMOR BOARD MEETING
Day / Date / Time / Location

OPERATED CASES

Case

MRN		Age		Menop		MS		F/H		G	P	Gender	
Medical oncologist				**Breast surgeon**				**Radiation oncologist**					
History		Breast disease checklist — History of breast surgery type/date, chemotherapy type/cycles and radiation											
Combined Breast Clinic Date		Seen first time in combined breast clinic											
Combined Breast Clinic physical Examination													
Tumor board conference date													
Conference Decision													
Pre op Treatment		Type of Neoadjuvant treatment, number of cycles											
Clinical/radiological Response		Complete or partial response, stable or progressive disease											
Pre op Examination		Clinical examination before surgery											
Biopsy breast +/- axilla		Type of cancer in breast				**CT Chest**							
Mammogram						**CT Abdomen**							
Breast US						**Bone Scan**							
						Stage		T N M					
Surgery		Type and date of surgery (intraoperative result)											
Final Pathology						**Non-Invasive**				**Grade**			
Tumor Size		**Margins**				**Lymph-Vascular Invasion**							
LN Positive		**LN Removed**				**Extra-nodal Extension**							
ER		**PR**				**HER2**				**KI 67**			
Form is filled by													
Comment													
Decision		Post-surgery decision as adjuvant treatment or need further surgery											

BREAST TUMOR BOARD MEETING
Day / Date / Time / Location

COMBINED BREAST CLINC

Case#

MRN		Age		Menop		MS		F/H		G		P		gender	
Date			Medical oncologist			Surgeon					Radiation oncology				
history															
Breast disease checklist															
History of breast surgery type/date ,chemotherapy type/cycles and radiation															
Physical examination															
Breast examination checklist															
Images and staging															
Biopsy						CT Chest									
Mammogram						CT Abdomen									
US breast						Bone Scan									
						Stage		T N M							
Pathology															
Pathology						Non-Invasive					Grade				
Tumor Size						Margins					Lymph-Vascular Invasion				
LN Positive						Removed					Extra-nodal Extension				
ER				PR			HER2				KI 67				
Comments															
Combined clinic orders	Combined clinic orders checklist														
Decision	Tumor board conference decision														

Menop menopause **MS** marital status **F/H** family history **G** gravid **P** Para **LN** lymph nodes

www.ingramcontent.com/pod-product-compliance
Lightning Source LLC
Chambersburg PA
CBHW040032110426
42738CB00048B/41